Ketogenic Diet

Ultimate Beginner's Guide to Healthy, Long Term Weight Loss

Michael Wease

Table of Contents

Introduction

I want to thank you and congratulate you for purchasing the book, Ketogenic Diet.

This book contains proven steps and strategies on how to successfully lose weight while on the ketogenic diet.

In this book, you will learn all about how the ketogenic diet works and how it compares to some of the other mainstream diets. You will also get a 30-day challenge guide along with 38 recipes to help get you started on your weight loss journey.

Thanks again for purchasing this book, I hope you enjoy it!

How Keto Works

A ketogenic diet is a diet that is extremely low in carbs and high in fats. It will allow your body to stop being dependent on carbs for energy and start breaking down fats into a chemical compound known as ketones to be used for energy.

How to Know You are in Ketosis

Your body does ketosis every day. It doesn't matter what you eat. Your body adapts and processes various nutrients into fuel. It needs fuel to be able to function. Proteins, fats, and carbs are all used. Consuming a diet that is low in carbs but higher in fats will increase the process. This chemical reaction is normal and safe.

When you consume large amounts of protein or carbs, your body breaks them down into a sugar called glucose. Glucose helps to create ATP. This is a fuel we need for our everyday activities and to maintain our bodies.

If your body can't use the glucose several things will happen to it:

Lipogenesis occurs if there is sufficient glycogen in the liver and muscles. The extra gets turned into fat and is stored.

Glycogenesis occurs when extra glucose is converted into glycogen and gets stored in your muscles and liver. Most of our daily energy is stored as glycogen.

Ketosis occurs when the body doesn't have any glycogen or glucose.

When your body doesn't have any access to food such as when you are on a ketogenic diet or sleeping, the body will burn fats and create ketones.

Ketones get created when the body starts to break down fats. These create fatty acids, and are burned by the liver. This is beta-oxidation. This results in the making of ketones. These are used as fuel by the brain and muscles.

To simplify, since your body doesn't have any glycogen or glucose, ketosis starts and your body uses up the fat that has been stored as energy.

Ketosis works when the fat gets broken down in the liver then the fatty acids and glycerol are released. The fatty acids are broken down even more in ketogenesis. The result of this process is called acetoacetate.

With time, your body expels fewer ketone bodies. You might start to think that the ketosis is slowing down. This isn't what's happening. The brain burns it as fuel so the body gives the brain the right amount of energy.

Your body needs glucose in small amounts to stay in good health. You do not need carbs. The liver will make sure it has plenty of glucose in the blood to keep your body healthy.

Most excess protein gets changed into glucose. Too much protein can be dangerous and stop the ketosis.

You need low levels of the hormone insulin. The easiest way to do it is eating a low carb diet or a ketogenic diet. There are other ways to increase ketosis, one way being to add in intermittent fasting.

How will you know that you are in ketosis? You can test it by taking samples of your breath, blood, or urine. Other signs don't require a test. These are:

- Increased thirst and dry mouth. If you don't drink enough water and get the required electrolytes, you might develop a dry mouth. Try drinking a cup or two of bouillon each day. Always drink as much water as you want.

- Increased urination. A ketone body, known as acetoacetate, ends up in the urine. You can test for ketosis using urine strips. When starting out, it can cause you to need to use the bathroom more often. This is what causes the increased thirst.

- Keto breath. This is caused by the ketone body acetone escaping with the breath. It makes the breath smell fruity or like nail polish remover. This breath might be bad for your social standing. Most dieters will just brush their teeth often or use gum to help. If you choose to use gum, make sure it is sugar-free and check for carbs, so it doesn't reduce the ketone levels. This smell can be noticed in sweat when you are working out. It is usually temporary.

- Reduced hunger. Most people will experience a noticeable reduction in hunger. This could be caused by the increased ability of the body being fueled by fat. It could be from the increased vegetable and protein intake and changes in the body's hunger hormones. Most people feel great when eating just a couple times a day. Which ends up being intermittent fasting. This will save you both money and time. It also speeds up weight loss.

- Increased energy: After a few days of experiencing the keto flu and feeling tired, most people will have increased energy levels. This could be a sense of euphoria, brain fog being gone, or having clear thinking. Ketones are a very potent fuel source for the brain. Ketones have been tested to treat brain conditions and diseases like memory loss and concussions. Long-term dieters report more clarity and better brain function. Eliminating carbs will help stabilize and control blood sugar levels. This will improve brain function and increase focus.

- Weight loss: Ketogenic diets are very effective for losing weight. You might experience both long-and short-term weight loss when starting a keto diet.

Rapid weight loss might happen in the first week. Most think this is fat loss, but it is just stored carbs and water. Once the initial drop in water weight is over, you will continue to lose body fat if you stick to the diet and stay in caloric deficit.

- The decrease in performance: As stated above, when hitting the keto flu, and feeling tired, this might cause a decrease in exercise performance. This is caused by reducing the glycogen level in your muscles. Glycogen is the main fuel source for high-intensity exercise. After a few weeks, most dieters will get their energy level back. For some types of endurance sports, a ketogenic diet might be beneficial. One benefit is the ability to burn fat while exercising.

- Insomnia: A big issue for keto dieters is sleep at first. Most people have insomnia when they begin reducing their carbs drastically. This should improve in a few weeks. Many long-term dieters say that they start sleeping better after getting adapted to the diet.

Side Effects

Just like any change to what you eat, it is normal to experience some side effects as your body adapts to a new way to eat. When you start a low carb diet and reach ketosis, it is normal to have some side effects your first week. These might include loss of energy, leg cramps, digestive issues, keto flu, and loss of salts.

- Loss of energy: Switching to a keto diet is a big issue for new dieters. A well-known side effect might include fatigue and weakness. This can cause people to stop the diet before they ever reach ketosis and begin to reap the long-term benefits. These are normal. After years of running on high carbs, your body is being forced to adapt to a different fuel system. This switch will not occur overnight. It might take anywhere from seven to 30 days before you are in full ketosis. To reduce the fatigue, you might want to take an electrolyte supplement. Electrolytes are usually lost due to the rapid loss of your body's water content and getting rid of processed foods that have added salt. When adding in electrolytes try to get between 2,000 and 4,000 mg of sodium, 300 mg of magnesium, and 1,000 mg of potassium each day.

- Leg cramps: Getting muscle cramps is a normal side effect of a keto diet. These are benign but could be bothersome. The main cause of cramps is a condition called hyponatremia. This happens when your sodium level gets low. This can be helped by the recommendations above on salt and water intake.

- Digestive issues: A keto diet involves a major change in what you eat. Problems like diarrhea and constipation are common at first. These should subside after the transition period. Try to take note of the foods that might be causing these digestive problems. Eat plenty of low carb vegetables. These are low in carbs but contain lots of fiber.

- Keto flu: The first weeks of transitioning to a keto diet is challenging for some. Your body is used to using glucose for energy, and it has to learn to switch to ketones. This process is called keto-adaption. This can result in some brain fog but disappears when the body had adapted, and some might feel more alert. This adaptation might take about four weeks, but the side effects usually disappear sooner. By the end of your first week, you might feel some symptoms similar to the flu-like cravings, insomnia, heart palpitations, fatigue, dizziness, and brain fog. You might find that easing into ketosis will lessen these effects. You can do this by gradually lowering your carb intake over weeks instead of days.

- Loss of salts: There will be some changes in fluid balance that will occur in the first few weeks on a diet. This happens when the body uses stored sugar, and that releases water into the blood that gets passed out of the body with urine. As stated above, this can result in the salt in the body getting depleted, also. Just remember to keep yourself hydrated and add salt and electrolytes back into the diet.

Perks of Healthy Foods

Most people try to lose weight by just focusing on cutting calories, eating a high level of carb, and reducing the fat content in the diet. This will give some benefits. Low carb diets help to get rid of hunger and boosts weight loss by changing hormonal levels. Diets that are high in protein and good fats are filling and can reduce overeating empty calories, junk food, and sweets. For most people that are eating a low carb diet, it is easy to eat the appropriate calories. Foods like snack bars, desserts, ice cream, cereals, bread, cookies, sugary drinks are a big no, no.

A keto diet can help people who have type 2 diabetes who don't take insulin or people wishing to reverse the condition of prediabetes. Low carb diets improve the dyslipidemia of diabetes and the risk factors of getting metabolic syndrome.

Low carb diets are beneficial in improving blood pressure, insulin secretion, and postprandial glycemia. People with diabetes who take insulin need to contact their doctor before starting a keto diet since insulin dosages will need to be adjusted.

Even though the keto diet is high in fat, studies show that eating like this doesn't raise cholesterol scores. It also doesn't increase the risk of heart disease. Heart disease is caused by inflammation and is influenced by eating unhealthy foods like too much processed foods, sugar, and trans fats. Eating heart healthy fats such as fish, nuts, and olive oil is beneficial for the heart.

Low carb diets that are high in plant foods, nuts, olive oil, and healthy fats can lower the risk of heart disease, obesity and decrease the likelihood of complications from these conditions.

Fatty acids like omega-3s and omega-6s are needed for cognitive function. Your body can't produce them on its own because we lack the required enzymes. They have to be consumed by eating them or taking a supplement. This is where the keto diet is beneficial. Studies have shown that the normal diet doesn't have the essential fatty acids like omega-3s that we need. Fatty acids make up the majority of the brain's tissues; they are important in how the brain functions. It has a direct link to sensory performance, memory, and learning. Research shows we need to supplement our diets with essential fatty acids but keep a good ratio of omega-3s and omega-6s. The ratio needs to be between 1:1 and 1:4 omega-3s to omega-6s. This is great for people on the keto diet since they consume lots of healthy oils that help to balance out this ratio.

Some people ask if they are physically active if they need to continue eating a low carb diet. The keto diet involves the dietary breakdown of high fat intake, moderate protein intake, and low carb intake. Eating low carbs puts the body into ketosis where the body makes ketones from fat that is stored to use as energy instead of carbs. This means that people who exercise while on a keto diet are going to be using fat as their fuel.

As stated, fat is used for energy when carbs aren't present. Carbs do provide more fuel so the body can perform at higher intensities. Fat provides the energy during exercise at low intensities.

Some athletes might require more energy quicker than others. A low carb diet is helpful with exercise for:

- Adapting the body to burn more fat.

- Maintaining a good blood glucose level while exercising.

- Losing more fat and improving health with regular exercise and eating low carbs.

- Performing low to moderate intensity levels of exercise with keto-adaptation.

- Preventing fatigue when exercising longer.

A low carb intake has some benefits for certain athletes. For example:

- Eating a low carb diet can be a good practice for off season athletes to keep healthy while resting.

- Exercising while the glycogen stores are low improves the function of fat usage, enzymes, and mitochondria to improve physical performance and health.

- A diet that helps with fat loss is great for improving the ratio of fat to muscle. This is critical for people who want to improve their performance or meet weight goals for their particular sport like boxing, weightlifting, and wrestling.

- Keto-adaptation leads to relying less on carbs while exercising. This helps athletes in events where there isn't access to food or for those who can't digest carbs during exercise.

- Research has shown that a keto diet can help to preserve glycogen stores and can prevent endurance athletes from crashing while doing their endurance exercises.

Some may argue over the benefits of a keto diet over a high carb diet for athletes. Ketosis for physical performance might be helpful for athletes doing ultra-endurance or low-intensity exercises to maintain health.

Other Benefits

A ketogenic diet can ultimately enhance your mood. Eating impacts your brain and that includes the parts that regulate mood. Even though there isn't one food that can act as an antidepressant, but maintaining your blood sugar with proper nutrition can help you feel better most days. Foods that are rich in minerals and vitamins like vegetables and fruits have been known to lower the risk of depression. Foods that are rich in omega-3s like fatty fish, salmon and nuts help with depression also. Eating healthy could contribute to reducing stress.

Keto and Cancer

Some studies state that keto diets starve cancer cells. A low nutrient, pro-inflammatory, highly processed diet can feed the cancer cells causing them to grow. Is there a connection between a high sugar diet and cancer? The normal cells that are found in our bodies can use the fat for energy. Cancer cells can't metabolically shift to use fat instead of glucose. A diet that eliminates refined sugar and other carbs might be helpful in fighting and reducing cancer. Carbs get broken down into glucose that feeds cancer cells. By taking carbs from the diet, it can deplete the energy supply for cancer cells.

Cancer cells vary from normal cells in several ways. One unique trait involves insulin receptors. There are ten times more insulin receptors on their surface. This lets the cancer cells gorge themselves in nutrients and glucose that is coming from the bloodstream incredibly fast. As you continue eating glucose, the cancer cells continue to spread and thrive. The lower survival rates in cancer patients are those who have very high blood sugar levels.

Cancer cells have damaged mitochondria that prevent them from working properly. They can't metabolize fatty acids they need for energy. Cancer cells love oxygen-depleted living conditions. This diet is effective if combined with intermittent fasting. Fasting will increase ketone production and starve cancer cells.

Fasting might involve a person eating only four to eight hours a day. A 16-hour fast involves eating food in an 8-hour window every day. This lifestyle allows the body to produce ketones that fuel the whole body. This fast is optimal for people who have been diagnosed with cancer but can be incorporated into any lifestyle by using a 16 to 18 hour fast.

Eating a keto diet isn't the only way you can lower your cancer risk. Believers of the keto diet think that this diet needs to be prescribed for anyone who has a family history of cancer or is at a high risk of developing this dreaded disease.

History of Ketogenic

The keto diet gained popularity as a therapy for epilepsy in the 1920s. It provided an alternative to fasting, which had some success as a treatment for epilepsy. This was abandoned because of the introduction of anticonvulsant medication. Most cases of epilepsy might be controlled with medication. They fail to achieve control in about 30 percent of people with epilepsy. For those, particularly children who have epilepsy, this diet was introduced as a technique to help manage it.

Fasting and the treatment of this disease have been around for thousands of years. It was studied by ancient Greek and Indian physicians. An entry in the Hippocratic Corpus tells how changes in the diet played a role in managing epilepsy. The same author describes a man that was cured when he stopped consuming food and drink.

The first scientific study introducing fasting as a cure for epilepsy was done in France in the year 1911. During this time, potassium bromide was being used to treat epilepsy, but this slowed down patient's mental capabilities. Twenty patients followed a low calorie, vegetarian diet combined with fasting. Two patients had major improvements, although some could not stick to the dietary plan. The diet improved patient's mental abilities as compared with the ones who took potassium bromide.

In 1921, Rollin Woodyatt noticed that ketones were produced by the liver caused by starvation or eating a diet rich in fats and low in carbs. He called this the ketogenic diet and used it to treat epilepsy in 1921. In 1971, Peter Huttenlocher developed a keto diet where 60 percent of the calories were from MCT oil that allowed more carbs and protein to be included as compared with the original diet. This meant that parents could fix meals that were more enjoyable for children with epilepsy. Many hospitals have adopted the MCT diet instead of the keto diet although some use a combination of the two.

Going Out

It doesn't matter if you are out and need a quick meal, or you want to have a sit-down meal with the family, you should be able to find keto friendly foods at most restaurants.

There are plenty of keto restaurant options. Here are some rules that you can apply to almost any food place:

- Stick to vegetables, cheese, and meat: Most restaurants put extra carbs and sugar in their ingredients. Just stick to simple ingredients.

- Stay away from the bun: If you want a burger, you can choose to leave off the bun. You can usually add extra sides like sauces, bacon, and avocado.

- If you choose a salad, look at the ingredients: Most salads have leafy greens and berries that are high in carbs. Stick to simple salads that include meat and get the dressing on the side. Most Greek restaurants have low carb gyro salads. Stay away from croutons if possible and pick out the extra items that have carbs.

- Avoid it if it's breaded: Most fried items, mozzarella sticks, and chicken wings are breaded with some sort of flour-based breading. If there aren't any other options, peel off the breading. Pair the naked meat with a fatty sauce.

- Watch out for the condiments: While dressings and sauces are a great way to get flavor and fat into your food, but they are filled with sugar. Be careful of any sweet tasting sauces. Opt for fattier salad dressing like bleu cheese, Caesar, and ranch.

- Special requests: Some people don't like asking for certain foods, you can at higher quality restaurants. Menus do a great job of telling you what each dish has in it. You can also request that the meal is prepared a certain way (low carb, gluten-free, etc.).

- If you don't know, just skip it: If you find you are stalling in your weight loss, the main reason might be you are not keeping track of what you are eating. There are many hidden carbs and sugars in foods that you consume that you have to watch what you order. Just a teaspoon of a sweet sauce can be 15g or carbohydrates, and that is almost your whole daily allowance.

- Check online: Most restaurants put their nutritional information online. Some offer a build your app where you can choose what ingredients you want. This is a great way to see exactly how many carbs are going to be in the meat and sides you order.

Alcohol

Being on a ketogenic diet and having a social life can be hard to do. There are carbs everywhere, especially in bars. Stop drinking beer and wine is the first step but hard liquor is your best choice. Yes, hard liquor is made from fruits, potatoes, grains, and sugars but during the fermentation process, sugar is converted into ethyl alcohol.

Drinking liquor can deepen your ketosis but might slow down weight loss. Ingesting alcohol effects the liver metabolism. This means that more ketones are made, the more you drink. When the liver is taking care of the alcohol, it is being converted into triglycerides that can positively affect the ketone production.

Many people experience getting drunk faster than normal. That might be great for some; you have to be careful especially when driving. NEVER DRINK AND DRIVE. If you are on a ketogenic diet, be careful when consuming alcohol.

Other people experience worse hangovers, so be sure to stay hydrated. Drink one glass of water per 1 shot of alcohol.

Here is a list of what you can drink while on a low carb diet. Try not to stray from this list if at all possible:

- Beer: Michelob Ultra, Miller 64, and Bud Select. Most beers are high in carbs, so they have to be avoided. Lighter beers have their nutrition information online so you can check before you go.

- Wine: Unflavored and unsweetened champagne, dry white and red wine. These are the lowest carb wines that you should consume. These range around 5 g net carbs per 5 oz. glass. Just be careful.

- Liquor: Whiskey, tequila, gin, rum, vodka. All unflavored and unsweetened liquor has 0 g net carbs. Most mixers and liqueurs have carbs so stay away from them.

All of the nutrition information is based on a serving size of one bottle or can of beer, a five-ounce glass of wine, and a 1.5 ounce shot of liquor.

Good and Bad Foods

Starting a new diet can be hard. Here are the most common foods and how to consume them.

- Eat what you want
  - Wild and grass-fed animal sources
  - Healthy fats
    - Saturated
      - Coconut oil
      - Butter
      - Clarified butter
      - Goose fat
      - Duck fat
      - Chicken fat
      - Tallow
      - Lard
    - Monounsaturated
      - Olive oil
      - Macadamia
      - Avocado
    - Polyunsaturated omega 3's from animal sources
  - Non-starchy vegetables
    - Bamboo shoots
    - Summer squashes

- Cucumber
- Asparagus
- Celery stalk
- Radishes
- Kohlrabi
- Cruciferous vegetables (dark leaf)
- Leafy greens
- Fruits
  - Avocado
- Condiments and beverages
  - Whey protein
  - Egg white protein
  - Gelatin
  - All herbs and spices
  - Lemon and lime zest and juice
  - Mayo
  - Mustard
  - Pesto
  - Bone broth
  - Pickles
  - Fermented foods
  - Pork rinds
  - Water
  - Coffee
  - Tea (herbal, black)

- Enjoy sometimes
  - Fruits and veggies
    - Olives
    - Rhubarb
    - Coconut
    - Berries
    - Sea vegetables
    - Okra
    - Water chestnuts
    - Artichokes
    - Wax beans
    - Sugar peas
    - Some root veggies
    - Winter squash
    - Mushrooms
    - Garlic
    - Onion
    - Leek
    - Spring onion
    - Nightshades
    - Rutabaga
    - Turnips
    - Fennel
    - Brussels sprouts
    - Broccoli

- Cauliflower
- All cabbages
- Grain-fed animal sources and dairy
  - Bacon
  - Dairy products
  - Beef
  - Poultry
- Seeds and nuts
  - Brazil nuts
  - Pumpkin seeds
  - Hemp seeds
  - Sesame seeds
  - Flaxseed
  - Pine nuts
  - Sunflower seeds
  - Hazelnuts
  - Walnuts
  - Almonds
  - Pecans
  - Macadamia nuts
- Condiments
  - Carob and cocoa powder
  - Extra dark chocolate
  - Sugar-free tomato products
  - "Zero-carb" sweeteners

- Average carb food
  - Tiny amount of – figs, pears, cherries, plums, orange, kiwi berries, kiwi, grapefruit, apple, nectarine, peach, dragonfruit, apricot
    - Chestnuts
    - Cashews
    - Pistachios
    - Melons
  - Root vegetables
  - Alcohol
    - Unsweetened spirits
    - Dry white and red wine
      - BAD
- All grains and anything made from grains
- Factory-farmed fish and pork
- Processed foods
- Artificial sweeteners
  - Saccharin, Sucralose, acesulfame, aspartame, etc
- Refined oil and fats
- "Diet" foods
- Sweet and alcoholic drinks
- Tropical fruit (banana, pineapple, etc.)

30-Day Challenge

This is an easy 30-day challenge that will help get you started. All the meals in this are listed in the next chapter and hyperlinked for your convenience. Some meals I tell you to eat leftovers. It makes for an easier day, and not as much cooking and waste. This is very flexible, so if you want to change something up and pick a different recipe below that I didn't use, then go right ahead.

With breakfast, you can choose a recipe you like and eat it every day, or you can just have coffee and skip breakfasts. This will save time, and also help you stay in ketosis.

You'll also need to figure out your daily calories and carbs and make sure you reach them no matter what the challenge says. Calories depend on what your current weight is now. Carbohydrates, in general, should be below 60 grams a day, but it depends on your body and how quickly you reach ketosis. If you are looking to lose weight instead of maintaining, then you should start below 30 grams.

Make sure you keep you cheat days at zero during this challenge; otherwise you're going to have a hard time. Once you have become used to this diet, you can get by with the occasional cheat day, but not in the first 30-days.

During this time, start listening to your body, and learn to stop eating when you feel full. Make sure you have zero carb snacks if you start feeling hungry between meals, and make sure you drink plenty of water.

Here is your basic 30-Day challenge.

Day One:

Breakfast: Chili Cheese Muffins

Lunch: Chili Turkey Burgers

Dinner: Mac and Cheese Casserole

Day Two:

Breakfast: Power Smoothie

Lunch: Leftovers from yesterday's dinner

Dinner: Stir Fry

Day Three:

Breakfast: Scrambled eggs

Lunch: Asparagus Basil Salad

Dinner: Mushroom Soup

Day Four:

Breakfast: Porridge

Lunch: Garden Dog

Dinner: Salmon Burgers

Day Five:

Breakfast: Crepes

Lunch: Spicy Slaw

Dinner: Roasted Chicken

Day Six:

Breakfast: Green Eggs

Lunch: Fish Sticks

Dinner: Chicken with Cauliflower

Day Seven:

Breakfast: Scrambled eggs

Lunch: Green Soup

Dinner: Leftovers from any previous day

Day Eight:

Breakfast: Chili Cheese Muffins

Lunch: Thai Chicken Wraps

Dinner: Shepherd's Pie

Day Nine:

Breakfast: Pizza Muffin

Lunch: Chipotle Lime Salmon

Dinner: Beef Brisket

Day Ten:

Breakfast: Power Smoothie

Lunch: Kaleslaw

Dinner: Curried Shrimp

Day Eleven:

Breakfast: Scrambled eggs

Lunch: Sesame Kelp Noodles

Dinner: Mustard Lime Chicken

Day Twelve:

Breakfast: Crepes

Lunch: Asparagus Basil Salad

Dinner: Chicken and Rice

Day Thirteen:

Breakfast: Green Eggs

Lunch: Chipotle Lime Salmon

Dinner: Cod Piccata

Day Fourteen:

Breakfast: Power Smoothie

Lunch: Leftovers from previous days

Dinner: Gefilte Fish

Day Fifteen:

Breakfast: Green Eggs

Lunch: No-Potato Salad

Dinner: Salmon Burgers

Day Sixteen:

Breakfast: Scrambled eggs

Lunch: Green Soup

Dinner: Stuffed Peppers

Day Seventeen:

Breakfast: Chili Cheese Muffins

Lunch: Thai Chicken Wraps

Dinner: Chicken Piccata

Day Eighteen:

Breakfast: Leftovers from previous breakfasts

Lunch: Stir Fry

Dinner: Lemon Chicken

Day Nineteen:

Breakfast: Crepes

Lunch: Spicy Slaw

Dinner: Chili Turkey Burgers

Day Twenty:

Breakfast: Chili Cheese Muffins

Lunch: Garden Dog

Dinner: Mac and Cheese Casserole

Day Twenty-One:

Breakfast: Scrambled eggs

Lunch: Fish Sticks

Dinner: Leftovers

Day Twenty-Two:

Breakfast: Power Smoothie

Lunch: Mustard Lime Chicken

Dinner: Beef Brisket

Day Twenty-Three:

Breakfast: Pizza Muffin

Lunch: Garden Dog

Dinner: Salmon Burgers

Day Twenty-Four:

Breakfast: Crepes

Lunch: Asparagus Basil Salad

Dinner: Cod Piccata

Day Twenty-Five:

Breakfast: Green Eggs

Lunch: Curried Shrimp

Dinner: Meatballs

Day Twenty-Six:

Breakfast: Scrambled eggs

Lunch: Gefilte Fish

Dinner: Broccoli Soup

Day Twenty-Seven:

Breakfast: Porridge

Lunch: Thai Chicken Wraps

Dinner: Sesame Kelp Noodles

Day Twenty-Eight:

Breakfast: Chili Cheese Muffins

Lunch: Leftovers

Dinner: Thyme Salmon

Day Twenty-Nine:

Breakfast: Scrambled eggs

Lunch: Chicken Parmesan

Dinner: Mustard Lime Chicken

Day Thirty:

Breakfast: Power Smoothie

Lunch: Garden Dog

Dinner: Leftovers

Recipes

Breakfast

Chili Cheese Muffins

Ingredients:

½ tsp sea salt

2 C packed cheddar cheese

1 ¼ C almond flour

2 tbsp red pepper flakes

3 eggs

½ tsp baking soda

Instructions:

Mix the baking soda, flour, and salt in a food processor. Pulse the eggs in until they are fully mixed. Pulse in the cheese and a tablespoon of the pepper flakes. Line a muffin tin with paper cups and scoop in a quarter cup of the batter into each.

Sprinkle with the rest of the pepper flakes. Your oven should be at 350. Cook for 25 to 30 minutes.

Pizza Muffin

Ingredients:

2-oz pepperoni

½ tsp sea salt

½ C parmesan

½ C cheddar cheese

1 ½ C almond flour

¼ C tomato sauce

4 eggs

½ tsp baking soda

Instructions:

Combine the baking soda, flour, and salt in a food processor. Add in the eggs, pepperoni, and both kinds of cheese.

Place liners in a muffin tin. Add a quarter cup of batter into every cup.

Your oven should be at 350. Allow them to bake for 25 minutes. Once done, top with a teaspoon of sauce, extra cheese, and pepperoni. Cook for another 15 minutes.

Crepes

Ingredients:

4 eggs

2 tbsp coconut oil, cooking

2 tbsp coconut flour

½ C water

1 tbsp coconut oil

Instructions:

Mix the eggs and flour in a food processor. Pulse in a tablespoon of oil and water.

Heat some oil in an 8-in pan. Place a quarter cup of the batter in the pan and rotate so that it covers the bottom. Once bubbles form, flip, and cook the other side until done. Place crepe in a plate.

Continue with rest of batter.

Porridge

Ingredients:

1 tbsp flaxseed

1 tsp cinnamon

1 C boiling water

1 tbsp chia seeds

¼ tsp sea salt

2 tbsp unsweetened coconut

¼ C walnuts

1 tbsp pumpkin seeds

Instructions:

Combine the dry ingredients in a food processor until finely ground. Pour in the water and blend; slowly moving from low to high, until it smooth.

Place in bowl and top with extra coconut, sunflower seeds, and raisins.

Green Eggs

Ingredients:

Oil

Sea salt

4 large kale leaves

4 eggs

Instructions:

Blend the salt, eggs, and kale until smooth.

Heat oil in a skillet. Pour in the eggs and cook until done.

Main

Chili Turkey Burgers

Ingredients:

1 tsp sea salt

½ C onion, chopped

2 tsp cumin

1 C cilantro, chopped

1 tsp chili powder

1 lb ground turkey

8-oz diced green chiles

Instructions:

Combine all of the ingredients together and form into eight patties. Grill until done.

Mac and Cheese Casserole

Instructions:

1 tbsp paprika

2 C cheddar cheese

½ C parmesan

1 tsp pepper

4 eggs

½ C heavy cream

4 C cooked spaghetti squash

1 tsp sea salt

1 lb ground beef

Instructions:

Brown the beef in a cast iron pan. Take off the heat.

Mix the eggs and cream. Stir in the pepper, paprika, and salt. Mix in the parmesan, a cup of cheddar, and squash. Mix in the cooked beef.

Pour everything back into the skillet. Top with the rest of the cheddar. Your oven should be at 350. Cook for 40 to 50 minutes.

Meatballs

Ingredients:

¼ tsp baking soda

½ tsp sea salt

2 tbsp Dijon

2 tbsp tomato paste

Shallot, minced

½ tsp pepper

Egg

1 lb ground beef

1 tbsp coconut flour

Instructions:

Mix the shallot, beef, and egg together. Stir in the remaining ingredients. Form a quarter cup of the mix into a ball. Place on a baking sheet. Repeat with the rest of the mixture.

Bake for 25 minutes at 350.

Salmon Burgers

Ingredients:

1 tbsp water

¼ C wasabi powder

1 tsp sea salt

½ C almond flour

1 tbsp lime juice

2 eggs

¼ C cilantro, minced

¼ C scallions, chopped

1 tbsp ginger, minced

1 lb salmon filet

Instructions:

Cube the salmon. Mix the salt, flour, juice, eggs, cilantro, scallions, ginger, and salmon.

Stir together the water and wasabi to make a paste. Stir the paste into the salmon mix.

Form into patties. Sauté patties in a skillet until golden.

Beef Brisket

Ingredients:

½ tsp sea salt

8 carrots, sliced

8-oz mushrooms, sliced

8 garlic cloves, sliced

1 tbsp garlic powder

Onion, chopped

3 C chicken stock

1 tbsp onion powder

1 ½ lb brisket

Instructions:

Mix all ingredients, except the meat, in a large crock pot. Nestle the meat into the mixture. Set for six to eight hours on low.

Stir Fry

Instructions:

2 tbsp ume plum vinegar

2 tbsp sesame oil

2 tbsp arrowroot powder

1 ½ C water

½ tsp sea salt

Zucchini, sliced

4-oz shiitake, sliced

2 heads bok choy, sliced

2 carrots, sliced

2 head broccoli

Onion, chopped

2 tbsp coconut oil

1 lb chicken breast

Instructions:

Cube the chicken. Place coconut oil in a skillet and heat. Place in the onions and sauté them until they are soft. Mix in the chicken, broccoli, and carrots. Cook 10 more minutes. Mix in the salt, zucchini, mushrooms, and bok choy. Cook another five minutes.

Pour in a cup of water and cover. Let cook for 10 minutes. Dissolve the arrowroot in ½ cup water. Mix into the veggies. Stir until thickened. Mix in the vinegar and the sesame oil.

Chicken with Cauliflower

Instructions:

5 garlic cloves, sliced

½ tsp sea salt

1 C black olives

¼ C lemon juice

1 lemon, zested

1 tsp pepper

Shallot, chopped

Cauliflower head, cut into florets

Bunch thyme

3 tbsp olive oil

1 lb chicken breast

Instructions:

Place the thyme along the bottom of a baking dish. Lay the chicken on top and sprinkle cauliflower over.

Combine all the rest together, and pour over top the chicken. Let marinate for at least an hour.

Your oven should be at 400. Cook for 45 to 55 minutes.

Sesame Kelp Noodles

Ingredients:

3 drops stevia

2 tsp ume plum vinegar

1 tbsp sesame oil

¼ C almond butter

Package kelp noodles

Instructions:

Soften the noodles in some warm water with a sprinkle of salt.

Mix the other ingredients and toss in the noodles once softened.

Mustard Lime Chicken

Ingredients:

¼ C Dijon

½ tsp pepper

½ tsp sea salt

1 tbsp olive oil

½ C cilantro, chopped

½ C lime juice

1 tbsp chili powder

1 lb chicken breast

Instructions:

Pulse everything, minus the chicken, in a food processor. Place the chicken in a baking dish. Cover chicken with marinade and let sit for 15 minutes.

Cook for 22 minutes at 350.

Shepherd's Pie

Ingredients:

2 C carrots, diced

1 C chicken stock

1 tsp pepper

2 heads cauliflower, steamed

1 lb ground beef

2 C celery, diced

½ tsp sea salt

½ tsp paprika

2 tbsp olive oil

1 lb turkey bacon, diced

Onion, diced

2 tbsp olive oil

Instructions:

Heat a skillet with oil. Cook onion until soft. Mix in bacon and cook until crisp. Stir in celery and carrots, cooking until soft.

Add beef and brown. Season with paprika, salt, and pepper. Pour in the brother and reduce by 60%.

Puree the cauliflower with olive oil until smoother. Place in a baking dish and top with the mashed cauliflower.

Cook for 30 minutes at 350.

Salmon Burgers

Ingredients:

1 tbsp coconut flour

2 eggs

¼ C sesame seeds

¼ C scallions, chopped

1 tsp ginger, minced

1 garlic clove, pressed

1 tbsp ume plum vinegar

1 tbsp sesame oil

1 lb salmon

Instructions:

Cube the salmon and mix with the eggs, sesame seeds, scallions, ginger, garlic, vinegar, and oil. Mix in the flour. Form mixture into patties and cook until golden on both sides.

Gefilte Fish

½ C parsley, chopped

1 tsp pepper

1 C carrots, grated

¼ C dill

1 tbsp lemon juice

1 tsp sea salt

Onion, diced

2 tbsp olive oil

½ lb salmon

2 eggs

1 lb halibut

Instructions:

Chunk the fish and place in a processor. Pulse until ground, but not pureed. Heat up a skillet and sauté the onion until soft. Pulse the juice, pepper, salt, eggs, and onions into the fish.

Add in parsley, carrot, and dill. Let refrigerate for three hours.

Boil a pot of water. Shape the fish into balls and drop into water. Allow to cook 15 to 20 minutes. Place in a baking dish and let refrigerate until cool.

Roasted Chicken

Ingredients:

Onion, quartered

2 tbsp olive oil

Head garlic, cut in half

Lemon, halved

Bunch thyme

Pepper

Sea salt

Whole chicken

Instructions:

Your oven should be at 425. Clean the chicken and pat dry. Place in a baking dish. Coat with pepper and salt. Stuff with the garlic, lemon, and thyme. Brush with oil and sprinkle with more pepper and salt. Tie legs and tuck in wings. Put an onion quarter in the corners of the dish. Cook for an hour and a half.

Stuffed Peppers

Ingredients:

1 tsp sea salt

1 C cilantro, chopped

2 tsp cumin

1 lb ground turkey

8-oz diced green chiles

½ C onion, chopped

6-8 bell peppers

1 tsp chili powder

Instructions:

Mix the salt, chili powder, cumin, onion, cilantro, turkey, and chiles together. Slice the tops off the peppers and clean out the seeds and ribs. Place them in a baking dish.

Place the turkey mixture into each of the peppers. Bake for an hour at 350.

Thai Chicken Wraps

Ingredients:

Peanut sauce

¼ C scallions, sliced

1 C carrots, shredded

1 C broccoli, chopped

1 lb grilled chicken breast, diced

4 cabbage leaves, chopped

12 romaine lettuce leaves

Instructions:

Put a tablespoon of cabbage in each lettuce leaf. Add a tablespoon of scallions, carrots, broccoli, and chicken. Drizzle with peanut sauce.

Lemon Chicken

Ingredients:

Peanut sauce

1/3 C olive oil

2 carrots, grated

Head lettuce, chiffonade

1 lb chicken breasts

1/3 C lemon juice

1 ½ tsp thyme, minced

½ tsp pepper

1 tsp sea salt

Instructions:

Combine thyme, pepper, salt, oil, and juice together. Lay out the chicken in the baking dish and pour the marinade over it. Refrigerate for six hours.

Grill the chicken until done. Place romaine on the plate you serve it on. Sprinkle on the carrots and lay on the chicken. Drizzle with peanut sauce.

Thyme Salmon

Ingredients:

1 tsp sea salt

12 thyme sprigs

1 lb salmon

1 tbsp olive oil

Instructions:

Your oven should be at 500. Place thyme on a baking sheet and lay the salmon on top. Rub with salt and oil.

Turn the oven off and slide in the salmon. Bake for 10 to 12 minutes.

Chicken and Rice

Ingredients:

Avocado

Chili powder, cumin, and oregano to taste

1 tsp sea salt

1 lb grilled chicken breast, diced

4-oz diced green chilies

Cauliflower head, trimmed

1 C celery, diced

Onion, diced

4 tbsp olive oil

Instructions:

Place oil in hot pan and cook onions until soft. Mix in the celery and cook five minutes more.

Put the cauliflower in a processor and mix until it has the texture of rice. Place in the skillet and cook until soft.

Stir in the chicken and chilies. Mix in the chili powder, cumin, and oregano.

Serve with avocado.

Chipotle Lime Salmon

Ingredients:

1 tsp chipotle powder

2 limes, halved

2 tbsp olive oil

1 tsp sea salt

1 lb salmon, cut in 4 fillets

Instructions:

Your oven should be at 500. Rub oil on the fillets. Squeeze lime half on each fillet.

Sprinkle with chipotle and salt. Reduce temperature to 275. Slide in the fillets and cook 8 to 12 minutes.

Cod Piccata

Ingredients:

¼ C parsley, chopped

¼ C capers

¼ C lemon juice

1 C chicken stock

5 tbsp grapeseed oil

5 tbsp olive oil

½ tsp chef's shake

½ tsp sea salt

½ C almond flour

1 ½ lb cod

Instructions:

Slice cod into six fillets. Combine the chef's shake, flour, and salt. Dredge the cod in flour.

Heat two tablespoons of grapeseed oil and all the olive oil in a skillet. Brown the cod on both sides.

Place the cod on a plate and put in a warm oven to keep warm.

Place capers, stock, and juice in the skillet and deglaze. Reduce the sauce and mix in the rest of the grapeseed oil.

Serve cod with sauce and parsley.

Fish Sticks

Ingredients:

1 C almond flour

6 tbsp coconut oil

2 eggs, whisked

1 lb white fish

1 tsp sea salt

Instructions

Slice fish into sticks, making sure to remove any bones.

Mix salt and flour in a dish and place the eggs in another. Dip fish in egg and then if flour. Heat a skillet with three tablespoons of oil. Put half the fish in the skillet and cook until browned on all sides. Place the rest of the oil in the skillet and cook the rest of the fish.

Chicken Piccata

Ingredients:

¼ C parsley

5 tbsp olive oil

¼ C capers

1 C chicken stock

¼ C lemon juice

½ tsp chef's shake

½ tsp sea salt

½ C almond flour

5 tbsp grapeseed oil

1 ½ lb chicken breast halves

Instructions:

Butterfly the chicken and then pound them to a quarter of an inch.

Combine the chef's shake, flour, and salt. Dredge the chicken in the flour.

Heat a pan with olive oil and two tablespoons of grapeseed oil. Brown up the chicken and slide them in a warm oven to keep warm.

Place capers, lemon juice, and stock into the skillet and deglaze. Reduce and mix in the rest of the grapeseed oil.

Serve chicken with sauce and parsley.

Garden Dog

Ingredients:

Sauerkraut

Dijon

Romaine

Hot dogs

Instructions:

Cook the hot dogs the way you like them. Put a dog on a lettuce leaf and top with mustard and sauerkraut.

Curried Shrimp

Ingredients:

3 tbsp lime juice

1 lb shrimp, peeled

Bunch cilantro, chopped

½ tsp turmeric

½ tsp coriander

½ tsp cumin

2 tsp ginger, minced

½ C tomatoes, pureed

Onion, chopped

4 garlic cloves

4 tbsp olive oil

Instructions:

Heat oil and add garlic and onions until soft. Mix in the turmeric, coriander, cumin, ginger, and tomatoes. Cook another five minutes. Add shrimp to the sauce and cook until done.

Mix in the cilantro and lime juice.

Chicken Parmesan

Ingredients:

16-oz mozzarella

6 sliced garlic cloves

1 tsp herbs de Provence

2 C water

14-oz tomato paste

6 tbsp butter

2 eggs, whisked

2 C almond flour

4 chicken breasts

Instructions:

Slice chicken into thin cutlets. Dip in egg and coat with flour.

Melt the butter and cook the chicken until golden.

Mix the garlic, herbs, water, and tomato paste together in the pan. Simmer for around 15 minutes. Put a half cup of the sauce in a baking dish. Lay the cutlets in the sauce and top with the rest of the sauce and mozzarella.

Cook for ten minutes at 400.

Extras

Spicy Slaw

Ingredients:

2 limes, juiced

Sea salt

7 drops stevia

1 tsp ginger, minced

Jalapeno, minced

2 tbsp olive oil

Carrot, grated

Bunch cilantro, chopped

½ purple cabbage, shredded

Instructions:

Toss all of the ingredients together and serve.

Asparagus Basil Salad

Ingredients:

½ tsp pepper

1 C basil leaves, sliced

½ tsp sea salt

2 tsp Dijon

1 C grape tomatoes, halved

2 tsp lemon juice

¼ C olive oil

Avocado, cubed

1 lb asparagus, trimmed and diced

Instructions:

Steam the asparagus until tender. Toss the avocado, tomatoes, basil, asparagus, mustard, juice, and oil together. Season with pepper and salt.

Kaleslaw

Ingredients:

¼ C almonds, chopped

4 carrots

2 heads kale

Instructions:

Slice the kale into strips and julienne the carrots. Toss everything together and top with your favorite recipe.

No-Potato Salad

Ingredients:

½ tsp sea salt

1 tbsp Dijon

2 tbsp mayo

2 hard-boiled eggs, diced

1 tbsp parsley, chopped

Small onion, chopped

2 celery stalks, diced

Cauliflower

Instructions:

Slice cauliflower into florets. Steam until tender. Let the cauliflower cool. Mix in the remaining ingredients.

Mushroom Soup

Ingredients:

½ tsp sea salt

2 qt chicken stock

1 lb shitake mushrooms, chopped

Onion, chopped

2 tbsp olive oil

Instructions:

Heat a stock pot with oil. Cook the onions until caramelized. Mix the mushrooms in, and cook until soft.

Pour in stock and bring to boil. Simmer ten minutes. In batches, blend in a blender until everything is smooth.

Broccoli Soup

Ingredients:

½ tsp sea salt

2 qt water

1 ½ lb broccoli

Onion, chopped

2 tbsp olive oil

Instructions:

Sauté onions in a pot until soft. Mix the broccoli and cook another five minutes. Pour in water and salt and cook for about 15 minutes.

Pour in a blender and puree until smooth.

Green Soup

1 tbsp lemon juice

2 qt chicken stock

2 tbsp ginger, minced

Bunch Collards

2 leeks, sliced

1 tsp sea salt

Onion, chopped

2 tbsp olive oil

Instructions:

In a large pot cook onions with oil until golden. Mix in leeks and cook another ten minutes. Stir in the ginger and collards until wilted.

Pour in the stock and cook another ten minutes. Puree the soup in a blender until smooth. Place back in the pot, heat, and mix in the lemon juice.

Power Smoothie

3 ice cubes

1 tbsp chia seeds, ground

1 scoop protein powder

5 drops vanilla stevia

1 tbsp almond butter

½ C kevita probiotic drink, coconut

1 C strawberries, frozen

Instructions:

Blend everything together until smooth.

Intermittent Fasting

Intermittent fasting is a great additive to your ketogenic diet. It will help you reach ketosis fasting, and help you to maintain it. It isn't another diet that you would have to follow, though. It's just your eating pattern. It helps you to schedule your meals in a way that gives you the most benefit. It doesn't have any effect on what you eat, but instead on when you eat. So why is it so effective?

One of the best things about it is that it will help you become lean without cutting down your calories. You try to keep your calories the same during the day when you begin intermittent fasting. This means that you would eat bigger meals during a shorter time period. The main reason why people start intermittent fasting is to lose fat.

To understand how this will lead to fat loss, you have to understand what the different is between the fed and fasted state. The fed state is when your body is absorbing and digesting food. Fed state normally starts after you eat and will last for three to five hours afterward. During this time it's hard for your body to burn fat because of the high levels of insulin.

After that, you enter into a post-absorptive state, which means your body isn't processing food anymore. This will last around eight to 12 hours. This is when you start the fasted state. Your body can burn fat a lot easier during this time because of the low insulin levels.

Since your body is only about to enter the fast state 12 hours after you last eat, it's extremely rare that the body ever enters this fat burning period. This is the main reason why you will start losing weight, without changing your diet, when you start intermittent fasting.

Benefits

There are other benefits to intermittent fasting other than fat loss.

1. It will make your day easier

Getting rid of one of your meals will make your life a lot easier. Whether you enjoy cooking and meal planning, or not, you're going to have a few extra hours to get things done. Instead of worrying about breakfast all you have to do is grab a glass of water or coffee and start your day.

2. You'll live longer

Scientists have discovered that reducing calorie intake makes a person live longer. This is because the body will find a way to extend your life when you're in starvation mode. Starving yourself doesn't sound fun, and it isn't something that you should do. Instead, intermittent fasting tends to have the same effect on your body that starving does.

3. It's easier than most diets

Diets typically fail because people aren't able to stick to it. Intermittent fasting stands out because it's extremely easy to implement after you get pass the fact that you don't need to eat all the time.

Conclusion

I hope this book was able to help you to understand and begin a keto diet.

The next step is to start the 30-day challenge and begin this new way of life.

Finally, if you enjoyed this book, then I'd like to ask you for a favor, would you be kind enough to leave a review for this book on Amazon? It'd be greatly appreciated!

Thank you and good luck!